The Ultimate LOW CARB Recipes!

Top LOW CARB Recipes for Beginners

Table of Contents

Introduction 1

Chapter 1: Getting Started with Low Carb Diet 3

Chapter 2: Low Carb Breakfast Recipes 5

    Cream Cheese Pancakes 6

    Bunless Cheeseburger 8

    Bacon Pancake 10

    Paleo Breakfast Burrito 12

    Flax Meal Peanut Butter Cereal 14

    Hot Pumpkin Cereal 16

    Almond Pancake 18

    Pumpkin Pancake 20

    Skinny Greek Omelet 22

    Low- Carb French Toast 24

Chapter 3: Low Carb Main Dishes 27

    Chicken Alfredo 28

    Lasagna in a Bowl 30

    Asian Noodles 32

    Poblano Pasta Salad 34

    Vegetable Pasta Soup 36

    Chicken Fajitas 38

    Chicken Marsala 40

BLT Chicken Salad 42

Chicken with Ham, Spinach and Pine Nuts 44

Chicken and Sweet corn Pies 47

Miso Chicken soup 49

Braised Chicken and Spring Vegetables 51

Chicken and Broccoli Cavatelli 53

Baby Back Ribs 56

Korean Beef 58

Crispy Pork Carnitas 60

Brined Pork Chops with Gremolata 62

Beef Lettuce Wraps 64

Swedish Meatballs 66

Hearty Beef Meatloaf 68

Steak with Potato Cauliflower Mash 70

Beef Curry 72

Beef Kebab 74

Tuna Casserole 76

Baked Salmon 78

Spiced Halibut on Tabbouleh Salad 80

Baked White Fish 82

Spicy Broiled Shrimp 84

Almond and Parmesan Baked Tilapia 86

Seafood Crepes 88

Cheesy Tuna Casserole 90

The Ultimate LOW CARB Recipes!

- Grouper with Crabmeat Sauce 92
- Garlic Lemon Shrimp with Cauliflower 94
- No Bake Cheesecake 97
- Microwave Lava Cake 99

Chapter 4: Low Carb Desserts

- Plain Biscotti 101
- Brownies 103
- Nutella Fudge 105
- Panna Cotta 107
- Spicy Baked Cauliflower and Sweet Potato 109
- Peanut Butter Mousse 111

Chapter 5: Quick Snack Ideas and Low Carb Snacks & Beverages 113

- Cheese Roll-Ups 115
- Nachos 117
- Peanut Butter Protein Balls 119
- Chocolate Nut Cake 121
- Shepard's Pie 123
- Black Bean Brownies 125
- Barley-Oat Chocolate Chip Cookies 127
- Nutty Carrot Cake Bar 129
- Asparagus Frittata 131
- Sports Drink 133
- Low Carb Iced Coffee 135

Strawberry Protein Smoothie 137

Iced Frappuccino 139

Chapter 6: Tips in Maintaining a Low Carb Diet 141

Introduction

I want to thank you and congratulate you for purchasing this book...

"The Ultimate LOW CARB Recipes"

This book contains various recipes that are guaranteed low in carbohydrate content so you do not have to worry about your blood sugar levels shooting up.

Low-carb diet is perfect for those who are also trying to lose weight and lead a healthier lifestyle.

This type of diet can jumpstart your way to a new and healthier you. It doesn't matter if you are new to this kind of diet – this book will get you ready for going low-carb!

Thanks again for purchasing this book, I hope you enjoy it!

CHAPTER 1

Getting Started with Low Carb Diet

A low-carb diet is a type of diet where, as implied in the name, carbohydrate intake is significantly limited. Food intake in a low-carb diet consists of those that have high protein and fat content. Aside from weight loss, a low carb diet has a number of health benefits such as lowering the risk factors of diabetes and hypertension.

Before starting with any weight lose regiment, consult with your doctor first especially if you have any existing health conditions.

Generally, low-carb diet focuses on high intake of proteins such as meat, eggs, poultry, fish, and vegetables that are low in starch. Foods such as breads, pastas, legumes, sweets, starchy vegetables, and grains together with some seeds and nuts must be avoided if you want to stick to a low-carb diet.

Low Carb Diet for Beginners:

To achieve success on this type of diet, here are some steps that you might find helpful.

Stay Informed.

Be familiar about low-carb diets. There are many myths about it so be sure that you are only reading from a reliable source.

Take Baby Steps.

As you are learning about low carb diet, you can start doing away with the unhealthy carbohydrates that you are eating. Reduce them little by little and you will be surprised with how easy it is to live a low-carb lifestyle.

Know the Healthy Carbohydrates.

Focus on the food that you can eat, not on what you can't. You can substitute a non-healthy carbohydrate food with a healthy one.

Plan Ahead.

Get a menu ready for at least a week. This will help you stick to your diet. Prepare your menu for the week and have an extra list in case you get delayed on planning the next menu set.

The first few weeks will be challenging. There are times when you will be tempted to go back to your old ways. However, understand that the feeling is normal. In order to be successful you have be committed all throughout your diet. Talk with people who have experienced doing a low carb diet and ask for their advice

CHAPTER 2

Low Carb Breakfast Recipes

Beginners may find it hard to come up with a low-carb breakfast. If you are used to eating cereal, bread, or oatmeal, then you are in for a surprise because you have to come up with a totally new breakfast plan. Below are some ideas for your breakfast.

Cream Cheese Pancakes

Nutrition Facts

Cream Cheese Pancake

1 Serving

Amount Per Serving	
Calories	341.0
Total Fat	29.2 g
Saturated Fat	14.1 g
Polyunsaturated Fat	2.8 g
Monounsaturated Fat	8.5 g
Cholesterol	434.0 mg
Sodium	310.1 mg
Potassium	221.7 mg
Total Carbohydrate	6.0 g
Dietary Fiber	0.6 g
Sugars	2.7 g
Protein	16.8 g

What you need:

2 eggs
1 packet sweetener
2 oz. cream cheese
1/2 tsp. cinnamon

How to prepare:

1. Blend all ingredients until smooth.
2. Allow bubbles to settle for about 2 minutes.
3. Heat a pan and grease it with butter.
4. Pour 1/4 of the batter on the pan and cook for 2 minutes until it turns gold.
5. Do the same with the other side.
6. Serve with sugar-free syrup and some fresh berries.

Bunless Cheeseburger

Nutrition Facts

Bunless Cheeseburger

1 Serving

Amount Per Serving	
Calories	1,045.4
Total Fat	70.2 g
Saturated Fat	37.8 g
Polyunsaturated Fat	4.0 g
Monounsaturated Fat	23.0 g
Cholesterol	217.6 mg
Sodium	2,395.0 mg
Potassium	1,119.0 mg
Total Carbohydrate	51.2 g
Dietary Fiber	4.8 g
Sugars	1.2 g
Protein	56.2 g

What you need:

Hamburger
Cheddar cheese
Cream cheese
Butter

Salsa

Spinach

Spices

How to prepare:

1. Heat a pan and put butter.
2. Add the spices and the burger.
3. Flip burgers until cooked..
4. Place cream cheese and cheddar on top of the burger.
5. Reduce the heat and cover the pan until cheese has melted.
6. Serve with spinach.
7. Salsa can make a juicier burger.

Bacon Pancake

Nutrition Facts

Bacon Pancake

1 Serving

Amount Per Serving	
Calories	615.4
Total Fat	46.7 g
Saturated Fat	17.5 g
Polyunsaturated Fat	2.4 g
Monounsaturated Fat	10.9 g
Cholesterol	92.2 mg
Sodium	985.3 mg
Potassium	171.1 mg
Total Carbohydrate	4.7 g
Dietary Fiber	0.2 g
Sugars	0.8 g
Protein	34.9 g

What you need:

5-6 slices of bacon
30 grams coconut flour
1/2 cup water

3 egg whites

2 tbsp. butter, unsalted and melted

15 ml purified granular gelatin

2 tbsp. chopped chives

How to prepare:

1. Fry bacon over medium heat and leave fat in pan.
2. Chop the bacon finely. Set aside.
3. Whisk egg whites using an electric mixer. Set aside.
4. Combine the gelatin, bacon, chives, and coconut cloud.
5. Add water and mix well with the egg whites.
6. Resulting batter must be thick.
7. Place some of the batter and form into small pancakes.
8. Top with bacon.

Paleo Breakfast Burrito

Nutrition Facts

Paleo Breakfast Burrito

1 Serving

Amount Per Serving	
Calories	103.1
Total Fat	3.6 g
Saturated Fat	0.8 g
Polyunsaturated Fat	0.1 g
Monounsaturated Fat	0.7 g
Cholesterol	14.3 mg
Sodium	563.1 mg
Potassium	99.2 mg
Total Carbohydrate	4.0 g
Dietary Fiber	0.4 g
Sugars	2.7 g
Protein	13.5 g

What you need:

2 egg whites
1/4 cup chopped vegetables
(olives, tomato, spinach, bell pepper)
Sliced ham, must be large and thick enough

How to prepare:

1. Heat pan and smear a bit of oil.
2. Sauté vegetables.
3. Whisk eggs ad pour over the vegetable mixture.
4. Scramble the mix until cooked.
5. Remove the eggs from the pan.
6. Roll ham around eggs and grill for a few seconds until ham is brown.
7. Optional: serve with cilantro, salsa, and guacamole.

Flax Meal Peanut Butter Cereal

Nutrition Facts

Flax Meal Peanut Butter

1 Serving

Amount Per Serving	
Calories	467.6
Total Fat	31.0 g
Saturated Fat	5.4 g
Polyunsaturated Fat	13.4 g
Monounsaturated Fat	10.9 g
Cholesterol	14.3 mg
Sodium	710.3 mg
Potassium	452.6 mg
Total Carbohydrate	20.7 g
Dietary Fiber	12.6 g
Sugars	5.6 g
Protein	29.0 g

What you need:

2 tbsp. peanut butter
1/4 cup flax seed meal

1/4 tsp. cinnamon, peanut
1/2 cup boiling water

How to prepare:

1. Pour water over flax seed meal. Stir well.
2. Add peanut butter and cinnamon.
3. Let the mixture sit for 1-2 minutes.

Hot Pumpkin Cereal

Nutrition Facts

Hot Pumpkin Cereal

1 Serving

Amount Per Serving

Calories	309.9
Total Fat	14.9 g
Saturated Fat	7.7 g
Polyunsaturated Fat	1.3 g
Monounsaturated Fat	4.6 g
Cholesterol	224.1 mg
Sodium	315.7 mg
Potassium	222.8 mg
Total Carbohydrate	23.9 g
Dietary Fiber	2.3 g
Sugars	14.0 g
Protein	21.1 g

What you need:

1 egg
1/2 cup ricotta cheese
1/4 cup pumpkin puree

A pinch of salt

Sweetener

Optional: 2 tbsp. seed meal

How to prepare:

1. Thin out ricotta cheese by mixing it with water.
2. Add egg and beat well.
3. Put in the salt and pumpkin.
4. Add sweetener to taste.
5. Stir under medium heat until it becomes grainy.
6. Add flax seed meal.

Almond Pancake

Nutrition Facts

Almond Pancake

1 Serving

Amount Per Serving	
Calories	542.7
Total Fat	50.6 g
Saturated Fat	7.8 g
Polyunsaturated Fat	4.3 g
Monounsaturated Fat	23.5 g
Cholesterol	372.0 mg
Sodium	142.0 mg
Potassium	138.0 mg
Total Carbohydrate	9.8 g
Dietary Fiber	3.0 g
Sugars	4.4 g
Protein	18.6 g

This low-carb pancake tastes better and it's also healthier.

What you need:

1 cup almond flour
2 eggs
1/4 cup water
2 tablespoons oil
1 teaspoon salt
1 tablespoon sweetener

How to prepare:

1. Grease a nonstick pan with a little oil.
2. Mix the ingredients just as you would mix your regular pancake recipe.
3. Flip the pancake when the underside is brown.
4. Serve with sugar-free syrup or any low carb topping.

Pumpkin Pancake

Nutrition Facts

Pumpkin Pancake

1 Serving

Amount Per Serving	
Calories	425.0
Total Fat	52.4 g
Saturated Fat	3.2 g
Polyunsaturated Fat	2.0 g
Monounsaturated Fat	3.6 g
Cholesterol	372.0 mg
Sodium	351.7 mg
Potassium	144.2 mg
Total Carbohydrate	60.4 g
Dietary Fiber	15.0 g
Sugars	26.8 g
Protein	15.9 g

What you need:

4 packets of Truvia

2 Large Eggs

2 tbsp. Coconut Flour
½ cup Pure Pumpkin Puree (canned)
1/2 cup Egg Whites (fresh)
1 tsp. Vanilla Extract
1/2 tsp. Double-Acting Baking Powder
1/2 tbsp. Ground Cinnamon
1/8 tsp. Salt

How to prepare:

1. Mix cinnamon, coconut flour, salt and baking powder in a bowl.
2. In another bowl, mix Truvia, pumpkin, egg whites, egg, and vanilla extract.
Then pour the dry ingredients over the wet ingredients and whisk together.
3. Use cooking spray over a flat griddle and place in heat.
4. Pour ¼ cup of batter on the heated pan until the center puffs and the surface bubbles.
5. Flip pancake and cook for 2 minutes
6. Serve with whipped cream, chocolate chips or maple syrup.

Skinny Greek Omelet

Nutrition Facts

Spicy Greek Omelet

1 Serving

Amount Per Serving	
Calories	183.9
Total Fat	10.0 g
Saturated Fat	5.1 g
Polyunsaturated Fat	1.0 g
Monounsaturated Fat	1.8 g
Cholesterol	206.0 mg
Sodium	409.7 mg
Potassium	276.4 mg
Total Carbohydrate	6.4 g
Dietary Fiber	1.9 g
Sugars	1.0 g
Protein	16.9 g

What you need:

2 tbsp. crumbled feta
1 egg white
1 whole egg
1 cup spinach
1 fresh basil leaf (diced)
1 tbsp. red onion (diced)
¼ cup tomato (diced)
salt and black pepper
Nonstick cooking spray

How to prepare:

1. Cook spinach and red onion on a frying pan.
2. Mix two tablespoons of water with basil, egg, egg white, salt and pepper.
3. Cook mixture on frying pan on low heat.
4. Spread the egg mixture on the pan by moving it in a circular motion.
5. Add spinach, tomato, feta mixture.
5. Heat until egg is cooked. Fold over, reduce heat and place in a serving plate.

Low- Carb French Toast

Nutrition Facts

Low-Carb French Toast

1 Serving

Amount Per Serving	
Calories	400.8
Total Fat	14.1 g
Saturated Fat	4.0 g
Polyunsaturated Fat	1.8 g
Monounsaturated Fat	4.8 g
Cholesterol	541.3 mg
Sodium	815.8 mg
Potassium	264.5 mg
Total Carbohydrate	41.1 g
Dietary Fiber	8.0 g
Sugars	4.1 g
Protein	34.1 g

What you need:

4 slices of whole low carb bread

2 eggs

1/4 a cup of milk

Sugar syrup

How to prepare:

1. Soak 4 slices of bread in egg and milk mixture.
2. Fry until bread is golden brown.
3. Place on a serving plate and sprinkle with cinnamon.
4. Pour sugar-free syrup and enjoy!

CHAPTER 3

Low Carb Main Dishes

Low carb meals need not be bland. Here are some main dishes containing low carbohydrates for you to choose from.

Low Carb Pasta Recipes

If you are a pasta lover then a low-carb diet would mean that you have to give up eating pasta. Wrong. There are many low-carb alternatives to pasta on the market that you can use.

If in case you wish to eat regular pasta, cook it *al dente,* so that it will not increase your blood sugar.

Pasta Sauces

You can use alternatives for pasta sauces such as spaghetti squash. They are even more nutritious and contain fewer calories.

When you are feeling up for some low-carb pasta, here are some recipes to follow.

Chicken Alfredo

Nutrition Facts

Chicken Alfredo

1 Serving

Amount Per Serving	
Calories	1,169.6
Total Fat	87.6 g
Saturated Fat	47.0 g
Polyunsaturated Fat	4.3 g
Monounsaturated Fat	31.0 g
Cholesterol	305.3 mg
Sodium	2,609.9 mg
Potassium	345.7 mg
Total Carbohydrate	10.9 g
Dietary Fiber	1.5 g
Sugars	0.7 g
Protein	84.9 g

This is a meal that can be prepared very simply.
To save time you can buy chopped vegetables, chicken and bacon.

What you need:

6 medium boneless chicken breasts
salt

black pepper
1 tablespoon cooking oil
1 cup whipping cream
4 oz parmesan cheese
1/3 roasted red pepper, cut into strips
Sauce:
1. Beat whipping cream in a medium saucepan for 1-2 minutes until thick.
2. Simmer under medium heat and reduce the heat after it simmers.
3. Whisk in cheese until it melts.

How to prepare:

1. Sprinkle salt and pepper on the chicken breast.
2. Using a nonstick 12-in skillet, brown the chicken evenly in hot oil for 10 minutes.
3. Pour the sauce over the chicken and top with sweet peppers.
4. Bake under 350 degrees for 15-20 minutes or until chicken is not pink anymore. Do not cover.
5. Add basil.

Lasagna in a Bowl

Nutrition Facts

Lasagna in a Bowl

1 Serving

Amount Per Serving	
Calories	426.4
Total Fat	15.1 g
Saturated Fat	6.7 g
Polyunsaturated Fat	0.4 g
Monounsaturated Fat	4.1 g
Cholesterol	37.4 mg
Sodium	931.8 mg
Potassium	96.6 mg
Total Carbohydrate	35.8 g
Dietary Fiber	10.0 g
Sugars	15.0 g
Protein	25.6 g

You'd be delighted to hear that you can still indulge in some; it doesn't contain a high amount of carbohydrates.

What you need:

1 lb. (serves 6) ground meat, cooked and drained
Makes 1 serving:

1/2 cup pasta sauce (sugar-free)
1/3 cup ricotta cheese
2 tablespoons parmesan cheese
1/4 cup shredded mozzarella
1 cup low carb pasta

How to prepare:

1. Cook the low-carb pasta.
2. Cook the meat. Add salt and pepper to taste.
3. Drain the excess fat.
4. Add sauce to cooked meat.
5. Heat the ricotta using a microwave to achieve desired results.
6. Arrange in bowl per layer: pasta, ricotta cheese, meat, mozzarella, sauce, parmesan.

Asian Noodles

Nutrition Facts

Asian Noodles
1 Serving

Amount Per Serving	
Calories	2,029.7
Total Fat	145.9 g
Saturated Fat	38.3 g
Polyunsaturated Fat	30.3 g
Monounsaturated Fat	68.4 g
Cholesterol	294.2 mg
Sodium	8,190.5 mg
Potassium	2,546.7 mg
Total Carbohydrate	68.1 g
Dietary Fiber	12.3 g
Sugars	20.2 g
Protein	114.6 g

Shirataki noodles are gaining popularity because they contain good fiber and no bad carbs. They can also have health benefits.

What you need:

2 tbsp. sesame oil

1-2 tbsp. mild oil

1 lb. ground pork

1 lb. bean sprouts

1/2 C soy sauce
1/4 C sherry (dry not sweet)
1/3 C peanut butter
1 tbsp apple cider vinegar
1/2 tbsp hot / chili sauce
2 tbsp grated ginger (must be fresh)
8 cloves garlic
6 chopped scallions / green onions
Pepper

How to prepare:

1. Mix pork, soy sauce, and dry sherry.
2. Set the mixture aside.
3. Mix the remaining soy sauce, peanut butter, vinegar, hot sauce, and add 1/4 cup water.
4. Heat skillet until hot enough.
5. Add mild oil or peanut to the pan and cook the pork. Make sure to break the pork into bits as you cook it.
6. Rinse noodles using hot water. Using a pair of scissors, cut them into shorter pieces.
7. Add garlic and ginger when pork is brown. Cook until you can smell the aroma.
8. Mix the noodles and sauce. Toss and heat through.
9. Toss again with bean sprouts and sprinkle with scallions

Poblano Pasta Salad

Nutrition Facts

Poblano Pasta Salad

3 Servings

Amount Per Serving	
Calories	353.8
Total Fat	17.2 g
Saturated Fat	3.3 g
Polyunsaturated Fat	0.4 g
Monounsaturated Fat	3.3 g
Cholesterol	3.3 mg
Sodium	424.4 mg
Potassium	92.7 mg
Total Carbohydrate	43.8 g
Dietary Fiber	7.5 g
Sugars	2.7 g
Protein	9.8 g

What you need:

4 ounces dried whole wheat rotini pasta

2 tablespoons snipped fresh cilantro

2 tablespoons toasted pumpkin seed

2 tablespoons red wine vinegar

1 ounce queso fresco cheese

1 medium red sweet pepper

1 medium fresh poblano Chile pepper

1 tablespoon olive oil

1 clove garlic, minced

1/2 of a medium sweet onion

1/4 cup chopped tomatoes

1/4 teaspoon salt

1/8 teaspoon black pepper

How to prepare:

1. Preheat oven to 425 degrees.
2. Slice Poblano and sweet pepper into half. Remove seeds.
3. Place the peppers and onions on a foil-lined baking sheet. Roast in oven for about 20 minutes until onion and pepper skin are lightly charred. After roasting, chop the peppers and onions.
4. Cook pasta. Rinse well with cold water. Drain thoroughly.
5. Combine cooked pasta and peppers, tomatoes, cilantro and pumpkin seed.
6. In a jar, combine vinegar, garlic, salt, olive oil and pepper. Shake well. Pour this dressing over the pasta and vegetables.
7. Garnish with a sprinkle of queso fresco.
8. Serve and enjoy!

Vegetable Pasta Soup

Nutrition Facts

Vegetable Pasta Soup

4 Servings

Amount Per Serving	
Calories	229.6
Total Fat	6.2 g
Saturated Fat	3.0 g
Polyunsaturated Fat	0.4 g
Monounsaturated Fat	2.3 g
Cholesterol	18.0 mg
Sodium	315.2 mg
Potassium	329.3 mg
Total Carbohydrate	36.4 g
Dietary Fiber	2.5 g
Sugars	2.3 g
Protein	8.1 g

What you need:

4 cups water

6 cloves garlic, minced

2 teaspoons olive oil

2 tablespoons snipped fresh parsley

1 1/2 cups carrots (shredded)
1 1/2 cups ditalini pasta, uncooked
1 cup onion (chopped)
1 cup celery (sliced)
1 box of chicken broth
1/4 cup Parmesan cheese, shaved

How to prepare:

1. Place oil in oven over medium heat. Add garlic and heat for 15 sec.
2. Add carrots, celery and onion for 7 minutes until tender.
3. Add water and chicken broth until it boils.
4. Add pasta and cook for 8 minutes until pasta is tender.
5. Top individual servings with Parmesan cheese and parsley. Enjoy!

Chicken Recipes

Always have a pack of boneless and skinless chicken on stock because you can easily create a decent and low-carb meal with it. You can have Thai for a night and Mexican with the other.

The Ultimate LOW CARB Recipes!

Chicken Fajitas

Nutrition Facts

Chicken Fajitas

1 Serving

Amount Per Serving	
Calories	273.5
Total Fat	8.0 g
Saturated Fat	3.1 g
Polyunsaturated Fat	0.4 g
Monounsaturated Fat	1.5 g
Cholesterol	108.8 mg
Sodium	2,127.9 mg
Potassium	56.7 mg
Total Carbohydrate	8.5 g
Dietary Fiber	0.1 g
Sugars	4.0 g
Protein	40.1 g

What you need:

3 lbs. boneless chicken breasts
1 tablespoon soy sauce
2 tablespoons apple cider vinegar
1 tablespoon Worcestershire sauce
2 teaspoons homemade chili seasoning (you can also use chili powder) frozen fajitas
1 slice onion, cut into strips
Optional: lemon juice

How to prepare:

1. Mix Worcestershire sauce, soy sauce, and spices.
2. Cut chicken into strips and place in a bag with the marinade. Marinate for 30 minutes.
3. Heat the chicken strips on the grill for 15-25 minutes.
4. Add the vegetables and cook for another 10 minutes.
5. Optional step: squeeze lemon juice.

Chicken Marsala

Nutrition Facts

Chicken Marsala

1 Serving

Amount Per Serving	
Calories	588.7
Total Fat	45.3 g
Saturated Fat	7.8 g
Polyunsaturated Fat	4.6 g
Monounsaturated Fat	33.1 g
Cholesterol	70.0 mg
Sodium	1,457.1 mg
Potassium	688.6 mg
Total Carbohydrate	13.7 g
Dietary Fiber	1.1 g
Sugars	2.4 g
Protein	28.4 g

A low-carb version of the chicken Marsala can be done with the use of dry Marsala wine.

What you need:

1 lb. boneless, skinless chicken breasts
1 onion (small)

1 cup mushroom slices
3 tablespoons olive oil
1/2 cup dry Marsala wine
2 tablespoons minced Italian (flat leaf) parsley
Chicken broth

How to prepare:

1. Season chicken with salt and pepper. You can pound the chicken if you want.
2. Add chicken on skillet with hot oil.
3. Cook chicken, remove from skillet and cover it with foil.
4. Add mushrooms and onions and cook until tender.
5. Add wine to pan and cook for 1-2 minutes.
6. If you want to have more sauce, add more broth and adjust seasonings.
7. Add vegetable and sauce over chicken.
8. Sprinkle with parsley.

BLT Chicken Salad

Nutrition Facts

BLT Chicken Salad

1 Serving

Amount Per Serving	
Calories	426.8
Total Fat	28.6 g
Saturated Fat	8.7 g
Polyunsaturated Fat	1.6 g
Monounsaturated Fat	4.4 g
Cholesterol	292.0 mg
Sodium	756.1 mg
Potassium	460.7 mg
Total Carbohydrate	4.7 g
Dietary Fiber	1.2 g
Sugars	2.5 g
Protein	34.3 g

Chicken salads can be topped with yogurt or mayonnaise. You can also add ginger if you want it to have a spicy flavor.

What you need:

1 boneless chicken breast (grilled)
½ small tomato

4 ounces of lettuce (chopped)

2 pieces of bacon (crumbled)

½ ounce of Swiss cheese

1 hardboiled egg (sliced in half)

2 tbsp. ranch dressing

A pinch of fresh parsley (chopped)

Pepper

How to prepare:

1. Grill the chicken breasts

2. Slice the chicken breasts into thin small sizes.

3. Arrange lettuce and chicken on a large plate

4. Add tomato, egg, cheese and spices evenly

Optional Ingredients:

Chives

Cucumber

Green Peppers

Avocado

Sunflower kernels

Chicken with Ham, Spinach and Pine Nuts

Nutrition Facts

Chicken with Ham, Spinach and Pine Nuts

5 Servings

Amount Per Serving	
Calories	443.7
Total Fat	31.6 g
Saturated Fat	11.5 g
Polyunsaturated Fat	4.7 g
Monounsaturated Fat	9.6 g
Cholesterol	43.3 mg
Sodium	889.4 mg
Potassium	746.1 mg
Total Carbohydrate	11.7 g
Dietary Fiber	3.0 g
Sugars	5.0 g
Protein	26.0 g

This dish is best served with white wine sauce.

Often served in restaurants, this Mediterranean Chicken recipe is an all-time favorite.

What you need:

300g spinach leaves

200g tub crème fraîche
150ml dry white wine
75g butter
8 chicken breasts (skinless)
8 thin slices of ham
3 tbsp. toasted pine nuts
3 shallots (finely chopped)
2 tbsp. raisins (chopped)
2 tbsp. olive oil
½ lemon juice
A pinch of spice powder
A handful of chives

How to prepare:

1. Heat oven for a few minutes.
2. Split chicken breasts, spread and bat out to flatten. Rub chicken with seasoning.
3. Place the spinach in a colander and boil with water. Squeeze as much water before placing it into a bowl.
4. Add spice and seasoning along with pine nuts and raisins. Combine and mix well.
5. Add a slice of ham over each chicken breast and cover with spinach mixture. Roll the ham and secure with a string.
6. Heat butter and oil in a pan before frying the chicken rolls. Roast for 10-15 min until cooked.
7. Add shallots with the remaining butter and cook until soft. Add

wine and lemon juice then let it simmer.

8. Stir the crème fraîche for 2 min. until thick. Add the chives into the sauce and stir lightly.

9. Remove strings from the ham then slice the chicken. Pour sauce around the dish and serve with potatoes.

The Ultimate LOW CARB Recipes!

Chicken and Sweet corn Pies

Nutrition Facts

Chicken with Ham, Spinach and Pine Nuts

3 Servings

Amount Per Serving	
Calories	463.0
Total Fat	29.8 g
Saturated Fat	10.2 g
Polyunsaturated Fat	11.1 g
Monounsaturated Fat	4.8 g
Cholesterol	85.3 mg
Sodium	688.5 mg
Potassium	86.9 mg
Total Carbohydrate	32.2 g
Dietary Fiber	1.2 g
Sugars	2.2 g
Protein	16.3 g

What you need:

500g puff pastry
6 tbsp. double cream
3 tbsp. Sweet corn

3 tbsp. peas
2 cooked chicken breasts (skinless)
1 tsp. Dijon mustard
1 egg (beaten)
Oil for brushing
Flour for dusting

How to prepare:

1. Heat the oven for a few minutes.
2. Roll the pastry on a floured surface and make rectangle cuts of about 24 x 36 cm.
3. Cut the pastry in half, and then cut each half into 3 squares of about 12 cm long.
4. Push each square into oiled tins pushing them into the edges. Push each square into the oiled tin, making sure it is pushed right into the edges
5. Cut the chicken into strips and put them in a bowl. Add peas, cream, mustard and sweet corn. Mix thoroughly.
6. Place equal amounts of mixture in the pies. Fold the top and press together so it can cover all the filling.
7. Brush the pastry with egg and heat in the oven until they are brown.
8. Serve and enjoy!

Miso Chicken soup

Nutrition Facts

Chicken Miso Soup

3 Servings

Amount Per Serving	
Calories	279.9
Total Fat	4.7 g
Saturated Fat	1.2 g
Polyunsaturated Fat	1.5 g
Monounsaturated Fat	2.1 g
Cholesterol	27.9 mg
Sodium	754.8 mg
Potassium	958.9 mg
Total Carbohydrate	39.6 g
Dietary Fiber	5.5 g
Sugars	16.1 g
Protein	18.5 g

Healthy Japanese chicken dish with miso soup.

What you need:

500ml chicken stock
50g long grain rice
8 Chanteney carrots
2 chicken breasts (skinless)
2 spring onions (sliced)
2 tbsp. miso paste
1 tbsp. soy sauce
1 tbsp. mirin

How to prepare:

1. Boil the stock in a medium saucepan for a few minutes. Add chicken breasts. Remove the chicken from the pan once cooked and shred chicken into pieces.
2. Add carrots and rice to the stock. Boil again and cover for 10 minutes until rice and carrots are cooked.
3. Place back chicken and add miso, mirin and soy. Garnish with spring onions before serving.

The Ultimate LOW CARB Recipes!

Braised Chicken and Spring Vegetables

Nutrition Facts

Chicken Miso Soup

2 Servings

Amount Per Serving	
Calories	382.2
Total Fat	11.1 g
Saturated Fat	3.2 g
Polyunsaturated Fat	3.1 g
Monounsaturated Fat	3.9 g
Cholesterol	231.6 mg
Sodium	818.9 mg
Potassium	1,393.0 mg
Total Carbohydrate	11.6 g
Dietary Fiber	4.3 g
Sugars	5.9 g
Protein	55.4 g

What you need:

12 medium radishes, halved
8 small bone-in chicken thighs

2 tablespoons chopped fresh chives
1 tablespoon olive oil
1 teaspoon sugar
1 cup low-sodium chicken broth
3/4 pound carrots cut into sticks
Kosher salt and black pepper

How to prepare:

1. Heat oil in oven over medium heat.
2. Season chicken with pepper and cook until brown.
3. Add broth, radish, carrots and sugar.
4. Place chicken on top of vegetables and simmer.
5. Cook for 15-20 minutes.
6. Sprinkle with chives, serve and enjoy!

Chicken and Broccoli Cavatelli

Nutrition Facts

Chicken and Broccoli Cavatelli

3 Servings

Amount Per Serving	
Calories	263.3
Total Fat	7.4 g
Saturated Fat	2.2 g
Polyunsaturated Fat	0.0 g
Monounsaturated Fat	0.0 g
Cholesterol	30.0 mg
Sodium	631.7 mg
Potassium	71.7 mg
Total Carbohydrate	33.0 g
Dietary Fiber	0.0 g
Sugars	2.2 g
Protein	16.0 g

What you need:

6 ounces dried cavatelli

3 teaspoons olive oil
3 tablespoons all-purpose flour
3 tablespoons butter
3 cups Broccoli spears
2 tablespoons Parmesan cheese
2 ounces pancetta
2 tablespoons snipped fresh chives
1 cup fat-free milk
1 whole bulb garlic
1 pound chicken breast (skinless, boneless)
1/2 teaspoon salt
1/2 cup evaporated fat-free milk
1/4 teaspoon ground black pepper
Snipped fresh chives

How to prepare:

1. Preheat oven to 400 degrees F.
2. Cut top of the garlic bulb to expose its cloves. Place garlic bulb on a foil. Drizzle with olive oil. Cover and fold the edges. Roast for 25 minutes until garlic is soft. Mash garlic in a small bowl. Set aside.
3. Cook pasta and add brocollini for the last 4 minutes of cooking. Drain but reserve ½ cup of pasta liquid. Set aside.
4. Heat 2 teaspoons of olive oil in an oven. Add pancetta and cook for 7 minutes until crispy. Set aside.
5. Add chicken pieces to the oven. Cook and set aside.
6. Melt butter in the oven over medium heat. Combine mashed

garlic, 2 tablespoon of chives, flour, pepper and salt. Add evaporated milk until the mixture is smooth.

7. Add the parmesan cheese, cooked chicken, cooked pasta and broccoli.

8. Add pasta liquid and top with crispy pancetta. Add extra chives.

9. Serve and Enjoy

Pork and Beef Recipes

Baby Back Ribs

Nutrition Facts

Baby black ribs

1 Serving

Amount Per Serving	
Calories	374.8
Total Fat	25.1 g
Saturated Fat	9.3 g
Polyunsaturated Fat	2.0 g
Monounsaturated Fat	11.4 g
Cholesterol	100.3 mg
Sodium	527.3 mg
Potassium	269.5 mg
Total Carbohydrate	15.0 g
Dietary Fiber	0.0 g
Sugars	13.0 g
Protein	20.7 g

Baby back ribs are often laden with sugar.
Now you can enjoy one without feeling guilty.

What you need:

Baby back ribs
Sugar-free BBQ sauce
Diet cola
Salt and spice

How to prepare:

Braising
1. Rub the ribs garlic and chili powder, pepper, and salt.
2. Wrap loosely in a foil and seal the area at the sides.
3. Pour half can of the diet cola or you can also use white wine.
4. Place the ribs in a covered grill under low heat or on a baking sheet in the oven.
5. Cook for 2.5 hours under 350 F.
6. Open the foil and brush the ribs with your BBQ sauce.
7. Grill under medium heat for 10 minutes per side.
8. Serve with sauce.

Korean Beef

Nutrition Facts

Korean Beef

1 Serving

Amount Per Serving	
Calories	345.3
Total Fat	23.6 g
Saturated Fat	9.6 g
Polyunsaturated Fat	1.1 g
Monounsaturated Fat	10.5 g
Cholesterol	86.3 mg
Sodium	3,916.6 mg
Potassium	623.8 mg
Total Carbohydrate	7.3 g
Dietary Fiber	1.3 g
Sugars	2.0 g
Protein	24.9 g

This is an easy recipe to prepare. You can marinate it to as short as 1 hour and as long as overnight.

The beef can be grilled quickly so it does not take up so much time.

What you need:

Beef
Marinade for 1 lb. of beef:
¼ cup soy sauce
¼ cup chicken broth
2 tablespoons sweetener
2 tablespoons sesame oil
1 teaspoon black pepper
1 teaspoon fresh garlic
1 teaspoon fresh grated ginger
2 scallions chopped
Optional:
1 tablespoon sesame seeds

How to prepare:

1. Slice the beef in strips.
2. Mix the ingredients for the marinade and put the meat.
3. Preheat grill and cook the beef strips.

Crispy Pork Carnitas

Nutrition Facts

Crispy Pork Carnitas

1 Serving

Amount Per Serving	
Calories	298.8
Total Fat	11.7 g
Saturated Fat	4.5 g
Polyunsaturated Fat	0.9 g
Monounsaturated Fat	5.5 g
Cholesterol	80.5 mg
Sodium	51.8 mg
Potassium	679.8 mg
Total Carbohydrate	13.5 g
Dietary Fiber	2.2 g
Sugars	0.1 g
Protein	33.7 g

Carnitas is served often during weeknight dinners and large parties. It is best paired with salsa, avocado and sautéed pepper. Perfect for special occasions, this dish will satisfy your guests and loved ones.

What you need:

4 pounds boneless pork shoulder (chopped)
4 garlic cloves (thinly sliced)
2 tsp. of salt
1 onion (thinly sliced)
1 tsp. chili powder
1 tsp. cumin
1 cinnamon stick

How to prepare:

1. Preheat the oven to 350 ºF (177 ºC)
2. Mix salt, chili powder, and cumin and rub it all over the meat.
3. Cook meat with cinnamon, bay leaf, garlic and onion. Add a small amount of water but do not drown the meat.
4. Cook until meat is tender and the liquid is gone. Slice the meat on a cutting board and shred into thin strips using your hand.
5. Roast meat until it is dark and crispy.

Brined Pork Chops with Gremolata

Nutrition Facts

Brined Pork Chops with Gremolata

4 Servings

Amount Per Serving	
Calories	508.9
Total Fat	20.8 g
Saturated Fat	7.7 g
Polyunsaturated Fat	1.7 g
Monounsaturated Fat	9.2 g
Cholesterol	182.5 mg
Sodium	1,832.5 mg
Potassium	838.5 mg
Total Carbohydrate	12.9 g
Dietary Fiber	0.5 g
Sugars	12.6 g
Protein	63.6 g

What you need:

6 tbsp. sugar
5 cups water
4 thin slices of lemon peel

3 bay leaves (crumbled)
3 tbsp. kosher salt
2 tbsp. parsley leaves (minced)
2 to 4 thick-cut pork chops
2 teaspoons minced garlic
1 sprig thyme
1 tbsp. fresh lemon zest
1/2 tsp. coriander seeds (lightly crushed)
Olive oil

How to prepare:

1. Prepare the brine two days before cooking.
2. Place a cup of water in a pan. Add bay leaves, thyme, coriander seeds and lemon peel.
3. Let simmer before removing from heat. Then add 4 cups of water. Stir sugar and salt until they are dissolved.
4. Put aside the chops in a bowl or freezer bag with the brine. Refrigerate for one or two days.
5. Rinse the pork chops with water an hour before cooking.
6. Brush the bottom of a skillet with oil and set on medium heat. Place the chops in the pan when hot and cook until brown on both sides.
7. Remove the chaps and cover with foil. Let it rest for 7 min. while you prepare the gremolata.
8. To make gremolata just combine lemon, garlic, and parsley in a bowl. Sprinkle it to the pork chops before serving.

Beef Lettuce Wraps

Nutrition Facts

Beef Lettuce Wraps

1 Serving

Amount Per Serving	
Calories	511.3
Total Fat	24.6 g
Saturated Fat	9.6 g
Polyunsaturated Fat	1.4 g
Monounsaturated Fat	10.3 g
Cholesterol	85.1 mg
Sodium	103.6 mg
Potassium	1,514.9 mg
Total Carbohydrate	47.3 g
Dietary Fiber	11.6 g
Sugars	3.2 g
Protein	28.2 g

What you need:

12 leaves of lettuce

4 green onions (chopped)
2 garlic cloves (minced)
1-2 tbsp. chili sauce
1 tbsp. vegetable oil
1 tbsp. soy sauce
1 tbsp. rice wine vinegar
1 tsp. ground ginger
1 red bell pepper (seeded and diced)
1 yellow onion (diced)
1 lb. ground beef
1/2 tbsp. honey
1/4 tsp. salt and pepper
1/4 cup hoisin sauce

How to prepare:

1. Rinse lettuce leaves, pat dry and set aside.
2. Heat oil and add bell pepper and onion. Cook for 3 minutes.
3. Add ground beef and cook for 5 minutes. Season with salt and pepper.
4. Stir garlic, chili sauce, ginger, honey, rice wine vinegar and hoisin in a bowl. Cook until sauce is thick for about 3-4 minutes. Add green onions.
5. Spread the meat mixture in a medium bowl. Arrange the lettuce leaves around and serve.

Swedish Meatballs

Nutrition Facts

Swedish Meatballs

2 Servings

Amount Per Serving	
Calories	420.8
Total Fat	30.5 g
Saturated Fat	14.1 g
Polyunsaturated Fat	2.2 g
Monounsaturated Fat	9.9 g
Cholesterol	181.3 mg
Sodium	1,336.4 mg
Potassium	421.6 mg
Total Carbohydrate	15.1 g
Dietary Fiber	1.0 g
Sugars	1.1 g
Protein	21.7 g

Meatballs seasoned with spice and served with a creamy beef gravy. Often served as appetizers and paired with noodles.

What you need:

2 cups sodium beef stock
2 oz. light cream cheese
1 lb. lean beef
1 egg
1 small onion (minced)
1 clove garlic (minced)
1 celery stalk (minced)
1 tsp. Olive oil
¼ cup parsley (minced)
¼ cup breadcrumbs

How to prepare:

1. Sauté onion and garlic in a medium heat pan for 5 minutes.
2. Add celery and parsley and cook until soft for 3-4 minutes.
3. Prepare a large bowl and mix beef, egg, onion, salt, pepper mixture and breadcrumbs. Mix well until all ingredients are thoroughly combined.
4. Use the mixture to form meatballs with your hands (about 1/8 cup size).
5. Add beef stock to the pan while it boils. Reduce heat and drop meatballs in the broth. Cover the pan and cook for 20 min.
6. After it's cooked, set aside the meatballs in a serving dish. Blend the stock with cream cheese until smooth.
7. Let the broth simmer for a few minutes then pour the meatballs into the pan.
8. Serve over noodles or put toothpicks if the dish is for appetizer.

Hearty Beef Meatloaf

Nutrition Facts

Hearty Beef Meatloaf

2 Servings

Amount Per Serving	
Calories	515.7
Total Fat	36.2 g
Saturated Fat	14.4 g
Polyunsaturated Fat	1.8 g
Monounsaturated Fat	15.5 g
Cholesterol	128.0 mg
Sodium	252.1 mg
Potassium	957.3 mg
Total Carbohydrate	13.6 g
Dietary Fiber	3.0 g
Sugars	1.8 g
Protein	33.3 g

What you need:

12 oz. crushed tomatoes
3 lbs. lean ground beef
1 cup pieces or slices mushrooms
1/2 cup chopped green peppers
1/2 cup chopped onions
1/4 cup beef stock

How to prepare:

1. Sauté onions, green peppers and mushrooms.
2. Add beef broth to the pan and let simmer for a few minutes.
3. Set aside to cool. Mix beef and crushed tomatoes in a bowl.
4. Fold in green peppers, mushrooms, beef broth and onions.
5. Shape beef into loaves and bake for an hour until juices are dry.

Steak with Potato Cauliflower Mash

Nutrition Facts

Steak with Potato Cauliflower Mash

1 Serving

Amount Per Serving	
Calories	500.6
Total Fat	23.9 g
Saturated Fat	9.5 g
Polyunsaturated Fat	1.2 g
Monounsaturated Fat	10.2 g
Cholesterol	85.7 mg
Sodium	264.5 mg
Potassium	955.7 mg
Total Carbohydrate	44.0 g
Dietary Fiber	9.0 g
Sugars	1.6 g
Protein	27.1 g

What you need:

3 tablespoons cider vinegar
2 cups cauliflower florets

2 cups cubed russet potatoes

2 -4 tablespoons fat-free milk

2 tablespoons snipped fresh chives

1 pound boneless beef top sirloin steak

1 tablespoon honey

1 tablespoon olive oil

1 can tomato sauce

1 clove garlic, minced

1 1/2 teaspoons chili powder

1/2 teaspoon salt

1/2 teaspoon onion powder

1/8 teaspoon ground black pepper

1/8 teaspoon ground black pepper

How to prepare:

1. Heat broiler for 400 degrees F.
2. Combine vinegar, honey, tomato sauce, pepper, chili, and onion powder in a saucepan. Wait to boil, reduce heat simmer and uncover for 5 minutes until mixture thickens. Set aside.
3. Broil steak for 15 minutes depending on your desired doneness. Brush the steak with tomato sauce last 3 minutes of broiling time.
4. Combine potatoes and garlic in a saucepan. Pour water so much as it covers the potatoes. Wait to boil, and then add cauliflower. Reduce heat, simmer and cook until vegetables are tender. Drain well.
5. Mix with oil, salt and pepper. Use an electric mixer to mix thoroughly. Beat until the mix is light and fluffy. Stir 2 tablespoons of chives.

6. Serve the steak with potato-cauliflower mixture. Sprinkle with additional chives.

Beef Curry

Nutrition Facts

Beeff Curry

3 Servings

Amount Per Serving	
Calories	461.5
Total Fat	34.7 g
Saturated Fat	13.9 g
Polyunsaturated Fat	1.5 g
Monounsaturated Fat	15.1 g
Cholesterol	125.0 mg
Sodium	121.1 mg
Potassium	604.8 mg
Total Carbohydrate	4.8 g
Dietary Fiber	1.1 g
Sugars	0.0 g
Protein	30.3 g

What you need:

1 500 g ground beef

1 cup tomatoes (chopped)

1 small onion

1 tsp. ginger

1 tsp. coriander

1 tsp. cumin

1 tsp. garam masala

1/2 tsp. cayenne pepper

1/2 tsp. turmeric

1/2 tsp. olive oil

Dash of salt

How to prepare:

1. Slice onions and sauté with olive oil in a heated pan.
2. Add beef and cook until cooked.
3. Mix all spices and add while cooking beef. Add tomatoes last.
4. Leave in heat until curry is cooked.

Beef Kebab

Nutrition Facts

Beef Kebab

4 Servings

Amount Per Serving	
Calories	342.1
Total Fat	23.6 g
Saturated Fat	4.7 g
Polyunsaturated Fat	1.5 g
Monounsaturated Fat	12.7 g
Cholesterol	28.5 mg
Sodium	1,233.9 mg
Potassium	109.2 mg
Total Carbohydrate	22.6 g
Dietary Fiber	1.4 g
Sugars	19.2 g
Protein	11.4 g

What you need:

20 bamboo or wooden skewers
3 tbsp. red wine vinegar
2 cloves garlic, minced
1-2 medium red onions

1 1/2 lbs. top sirloin steak
1 large bell pepper
1 tbsp. minced fresh ginger
1/2 to a pound button mushrooms
1/3 cup olive oil
1/3 cup soy sauce
1/4 cup honey
Freshly ground black pepper

How to Prepare:

1. Prepare ingredients and mix in a bowl. Add meat last.
2. Cover and chill in the fridge for 1 hour.
3. Wash the skewers before grilling. Preferably soak them for more than 30 minutes in water.
4. Cut vegetables in chunks following the width of the beef. Carefully pierce the meat and vegetables into the skewers.
5. Paint kebab with marinade. Grill the kebabs for 10 minutes until meat is cooked.
6. Serve and Enjoy!

Fish and Seafood Recipes

Tuna Casserole

Nutrition Facts

Tuna Casserole

1 Serving

Amount Per Serving	
Calories	249.3
Total Fat	5.0 g
Saturated Fat	3.2 g
Polyunsaturated Fat	0.8 g
Monounsaturated Fat	0.9 g
Cholesterol	67.9 mg
Sodium	617.8 mg
Potassium	719.0 mg
Total Carbohydrate	14.1 g
Dietary Fiber	6.5 g
Sugars	0.0 g
Protein	40.7 g

What you need:

1 14.5 oz. can cut green beans, drained
6 oz. can tuna, drained

2 tablespoons parmesan cheese

How to prepare:

1. Mix everything in a small casserole.
2. Microwave until warm.
3. Do not freeze.
4. Can serve up to 3.

Baked Salmon

Nutrition Facts

Baked Salmon

2 Servings

Amount Per Serving	
Calories	416.7
Total Fat	22.5 g
Saturated Fat	3.8 g
Polyunsaturated Fat	8.1 g
Monounsaturated Fat	8.7 g
Cholesterol	125.3 mg
Sodium	172.2 mg
Potassium	1,213.3 mg
Total Carbohydrate	3.2 g
Dietary Fiber	1.0 g
Sugars	1.5 g
Protein	49.1 g

What you need:

1 lb. salmon or other fish fillet
2-4 tablespoons softened butter

Garlic powder

Salt

Pepper

How to prepare:

1. Grease baking dish and place fish.
2. Sprinkle with garlic powder, salt and pepper.
3. Spread a thin layer of soft butter on the surface of the fish.
4. Bake at 425 C for 6-12 minutes or check the thickest part of the salmon to see if it's cooked.
5. Check frequently to avoid overcooking.
6. If you wish to brown the top, place it under the broiler.

Spiced Halibut on Tabbouleh Salad

Nutrition Facts

Spiced Halibut on Tabbouleh Salad

2 Servings

Amount Per Serving	
Calories	250.2
Total Fat	4.1 g
Saturated Fat	0.6 g
Polyunsaturated Fat	1.4 g
Monounsaturated Fat	1.0 g
Cholesterol	29.0 mg
Sodium	245.3 mg
Potassium	1,839.8 mg
Total Carbohydrate	32.8 g
Dietary Fiber	8.9 g
Sugars	2.7 g
Protein	25.7 g

What you need:

1 1/4 cups bulgur
5 large plum tomatoes (diced)
4-6 ounces halibut fillets

3 tbsp. fresh dill (chopped)
3 tbsp. fresh lemon juice
1 large pinch cinnamon
1 cup fresh flat-leaf parsley (finely chopped)
1 cup seedless cucumber (finely diced)
1/2 cup scallion (green part only, finely chopped)
1/4 teaspoon paprika
1/4 teaspoon ground cumin
Virgin Olive oil

How to prepare:

1. Place bulgur in a large bowl and pour 3 cups of boiling water. Stir well and cover. For 30-40 minutes, let bulgur soak until tender. Drain in a sieve and transfer to a bowl.
2. Mix in parsley, cucumber, tomatoes, dill, juice and oil. Add pepper for seasoning.
3. Heat broiler. Spread oil on a baking sheet. Wash halibut and pat dry.
4. Arrange on a baking sheet with 1 tsp. of oil
5. Combine and stir cinnamon, cumin, paprika and salt. Use this to sprinkle over halibut.
6. Broil for about 4 minutes. Then roast until lightly cooked. Serve on top of tabbouleh salad.

Baked White Fish

Nutrition Facts

Baked White Fish

1 Serving

Amount Per Serving	
Calories	413.6
Total Fat	31.6 g
Saturated Fat	4.3 g
Polyunsaturated Fat	8.8 g
Monounsaturated Fat	4.8 g
Cholesterol	25.0 mg
Sodium	550.5 mg
Potassium	154.0 mg
Total Carbohydrate	23.4 g
Dietary Fiber	4.0 g
Sugars	3.9 g
Protein	11.5 g

What you need:

3 tbsp. pine nuts

2 white fish fillets (6 oz. each)

2 tbsp. Parmesan Cheese

1 1/2 tbsp. mayo (regular or light)

1 tsp. basil pesto

1/4 tsp. finely minced garlic

How to prepare:

1. Heat oven to 400 F. Then use olive oil and spray on casserole dishes.
2. Mince garlic and pine nuts into fine pieces. Mix together with Parmesan cheese, mayo and basil pesto.
3. Spread the mixture over the surface of the fish .
4. Bake for 10-15 minutes until fish is firm and crust is brown.
5. Serve hot and enjoy!

Spicy Broiled Shrimp

Nutrition Facts

Spicy Broiled Shrimp

1 Serving

Amount Per Serving	
Calories	256.0
Total Fat	2.8 g
Saturated Fat	0.7 g
Polyunsaturated Fat	1.1 g
Monounsaturated Fat	0.5 g
Cholesterol	442.0 mg
Sodium	635.0 mg
Potassium	569.1 mg
Total Carbohydrate	13.8 g
Dietary Fiber	5.1 g
Sugars	1.8 g
Protein	48.9 g

What you need:

2 tsp. Worcestershire sauce

2 tsp. virgin olive oil

1 lemon (sliced in half)

1/2 lb. shrimp (peeled with tails left on)
1/2 tsp. Tony Chachere's Creole Seasoning
Salt and Pepper

How to prepare:

1. Place the shrimps in casserole dishes in a singer layer
2. Once arranged, add the following seasoning in this particular order: olive oil, lemon juice, Worcestershire sauce, creole seasoning, salt and pepper.
3. Broil for 10 minutes until the shrimp turns pink. Be careful not to overcook. Larger shrimps may take twice longer to broil.
4. Serve hot and enjoy!

Almond and Parmesan Baked Tilapia

Nutrition Facts

Almond Parmesan and Baked Tilapia

4 Servings

Amount Per Serving	
Calories	173.0
Total Fat	4.2 g
Saturated Fat	1.4 g
Polyunsaturated Fat	1.0 g
Monounsaturated Fat	1.3 g
Cholesterol	136.5 mg
Sodium	525.0 mg
Potassium	404.6 mg
Total Carbohydrate	7.2 g
Dietary Fiber	1.7 g
Sugars	0.6 g
Protein	28.0 g

What you need:

4 Tilapia fillets
2 tbsp. Parmesan or Asiago cheese (grated)
1/2 tsp. garlic powder
1/2 tsp. fish rub
1/3 cup almond meal
1/4 cup melted butter
1/4 tsp. pepper

How to prepare:

1. Preheat oven to 425F. Use a non-stick spray for the baking dish.
2. Melt margarine and butter in a pan with low heat.
3. Mix Parmesan, garlic powder, pepper, mix almond meal and fish rub in a flat dish big enough to hold the fish.
4. Dip the fillets in butter. Coat both sides with the mixture.
5. Bake for 30 minutes until the fish is firm and coat is golden brown.

Seafood Crepes

Nutrition Facts

Seafood Crepes

4 Servings

Amount Per Serving	
Calories	123.9
Total Fat	3.1 g
Saturated Fat	1.7 g
Polyunsaturated Fat	0.3 g
Monounsaturated Fat	0.2 g
Cholesterol	125.6 mg
Sodium	433.2 mg
Potassium	103.1 mg
Total Carbohydrate	7.3 g
Dietary Fiber	0.1 g
Sugars	2.3 g
Protein	16.1 g

What you need:

8 ounces of small cooked shrimp

6 ounces of crab meat

5 light crepes
2 ounces Monterey jack cheese (shredded)
1 green onion, chopped fine
1 tbsp. fresh parsley (chopped)
1 tbsp. chives (chopped)
1/2 cup sauce
1/4 teaspoon dill
1/8 teaspoon cayenne
For the sauce:
3 tbsp. butter
2 green onions (chopped)
2 ounces Monterey jack cheese (shredded)
1 cup heavy cream
1 cup water
1/4 cup carbalose flour
a dash of cayenne
a dash garlic powder

How to prepare:

1. Prepare the sauce first. Combine all the ingredients listed.
2. Fill the crepes with cooked crab and shrimp meat and roll up carefully.
3. Pour the sauce over the crepes and bake 375° for 25 minutes.
4. Garnish with green onions and serve.

Cheesy Tuna Casserole

Nutrition Facts

Cheesy Tuna Casserole

3 Servings

Amount Per Serving

Calories	362.7
Total Fat	27.4 g
Saturated Fat	17.4 g
Polyunsaturated Fat	1.2 g
Monounsaturated Fat	7.9 g
Cholesterol	111.8 mg
Sodium	604.7 mg
Potassium	242.2 mg
Total Carbohydrate	5.0 g
Dietary Fiber	1.3 g
Sugars	1.8 g
Protein	23.6 g

What you need:

16-ounce bag frozen French cut green beans
6-ounce cans of tuna (drained)
5 ounce of cheddar cheese (shredded)
3 ounces fresh mushrooms (chopped)
2 tbsp. onion, (chopped)
2 tbsp. butter
1 stalk celery (chopped)
1/2 cup chicken broth
3/4 cup heavy cream
Salt and pepper, to taste

How to prepare:

1. Cook green beans in a medium pot. Drain well.
2. Sauté onion, mushrooms, celery with butter until it browns.
3. Add broth and boil until liquid is reduced by half. Stir in the cream.
4. Season with salt and pepper.
5. Add tuna and mushroom soup in the green beans.
6. Microwave the mixture until cheese melts.

Grouper with Crabmeat Sauce

Nutrition Facts

Grouper with Crabmeat Sauce

8 Servings

Amount Per Serving	
Calories	239.3
Total Fat	2.6 g
Saturated Fat	0.6 g
Polyunsaturated Fat	0.8 g
Monounsaturated Fat	0.5 g
Cholesterol	94.9 mg
Sodium	107.1 mg
Potassium	964.2 mg
Total Carbohydrate	0.3 g
Dietary Fiber	0.0 g
Sugars	0.1 g
Protein	50.2 g

What you need:

8 grouper fillets
2 tablespoons marinade for chicken
1 tablespoon seafood seasoning

1 tablespoon olive oil
1/4 cup lemon juice
For the sauce:
8 green onions, chopped
3 tablespoons all-purpose flour
2-1/2 cups half-and-half cream
2 cups fresh crabmeat
2 teaspoons seafood seasoning
2 large onions, chopped
2 garlic cloves, minced
1 large sweet red pepper, chopped
1/4 cup butter, cubed
1/4 cup minced fresh parsley

How to prepare:

1. Place fillets in a foil-lined baking pan.
2. Combine lemon juice, seafood seasoning, marinade for chicken and oil in a small bowl. Use this mixture to brush over the fillets.
3. Broil for 7-8 minutes until fish is cooked.
4. In preparing the sauce simply sauté onions and garlic in a buttered pan. Add flour and seafood seasoning in the sauce. Add cream and wait to boil. Stir until the sauce thickens.
5. Add crab meat and stir until cooked.
6. Place fish on a serving plate. Sprinkle with parsley.
7. Serve fish with crabmeat sauce and enjoy!

Garlic Lemon Shrimp with Cauliflower

Nutrition Facts

Garlic Lemon Shrimp with Cauliflower

5 Servings

Amount Per Serving	
Calories	131.6
Total Fat	2.1 g
Saturated Fat	0.9 g
Polyunsaturated Fat	0.5 g
Monounsaturated Fat	0.3 g
Cholesterol	177.3 mg
Sodium	324.0 mg
Potassium	247.3 mg
Total Carbohydrate	6.2 g
Dietary Fiber	0.9 g
Sugars	3.1 g
Protein	21.1 g

What you need:

1 pound shrimp (peeled and deveined)
1 small head cauliflower (cut into florets)
2 teaspoon ghee
1 tablespoon lemon juice
1 tablespoon ghee
1 1/2 cups chicken broth
1/2 cup full-fat coconut milk
1/2 large onion, diced
1/2 teaspoon garlic powder
1/4 teaspoon black pepper
1/4 teaspoon sea salt
1/8 teaspoon black pepper
1/8 teaspoon sea salt
Chopped parsley
Zest of 2 lemons

How to prepare:

1. Use a shredder or grating blade to slice cauliflower. Set aside.
2. Heat pot over medium heat before adding onion and ghee. Cook for 4 minutes until onion begins to brown. Add chicken broth, coconut milk, cauliflower, salt and pepper.
3. Increase the heat and wait for the mixture to boil. Let simmer. Cook until cauliflower is soft and liquid is cooked.
4. Sprinkle shrimp with lemon, garlic powder, salt and pepper. Make sure it's well coated.

5. Heat a skillet over medium heat. Add ghee. Place shrimp in a single layer and cool for a minute until they are golden brown.
6. Serve shrimp with cauliflower grits. Add lemon juice and parsley as garnish. Enjoy!

CHAPTER 4

Low Carb Desserts

You no longer have to skip dessert even when you are into a low-carb diet. The recipes below will satisfy your sweet-tooth cravings.

No Bake Cheesecake

Nutrition Facts

No Bake Cheesecake

5 Servings

Amount Per Serving	
Calories	368.1
Total Fat	34.0 g
Saturated Fat	17.0 g
Polyunsaturated Fat	2.3 g
Monounsaturated Fat	11.0 g
Cholesterol	94.7 mg
Sodium	178.7 mg
Potassium	158.7 mg
Total Carbohydrate	12.5 g
Dietary Fiber	1.0 g
Sugars	9.1 g
Protein	6.5 g

This low-carb and no-bake cheesecake is very easy to make and you can use a variety of toppings.

What you need:

1 cup heavy cream
1 almond pie crust
10 oz. low fat or fat-free cream cheese, keep at room temperature
2 teaspoons vanilla extract
1 teaspoon lemon juice
Sugar substitute

How to prepare:

1. Bake the almond piecrust.
2. Combine the cream cheese, vanilla extract, lemon juice, and sugar substitute. Fluff it up.
3. On another bowl whip the cream.
4. Get a third of the whipped cream to the cream cheese mixture.
5. Spread the mixture of cream cheese into the crust.
6. Smooth off and chill for 2-3 hours.
7. Use toppings to cover and then serve.

To have a crustless cheesecake, simply chill the cream cheese mixture in a bowl and serve in individual dishes with topping.

Microwave Lava Cake

Nutrition Facts

Microwave Lava Cake

4 Servings

Amount Per Serving	
Calories	135.9
Total Fat	8.4 g
Saturated Fat	4.4 g
Polyunsaturated Fat	0.6 g
Monounsaturated Fat	1.4 g
Cholesterol	5.1 mg
Sodium	52.3 mg
Potassium	28.8 mg
Total Carbohydrate	13.5 g
Dietary Fiber	1.9 g
Sugars	9.8 g
Protein	2.3 g

A lava cake doesn't have to be sinful.

What you need:

1 square cacao chocolate, slice in half
1 tablespoon butter
1 tablespoon heavy cream
1 egg
2 tablespoons cocoa
1 tablespoon powdered sugar (Truvia)
a pinch of salt

How to prepare:

1. Place the butter in a cup and melt it in a microwave for about 20 seconds.
2. Mix vanilla, egg, and cream well.
3. Add the cocoa, salt, and powdered sugar. Mix until smooth.
4. Cover them with plastic wrap and microwave on high temperature for 30-40 seconds or until it sets.
5. Cut a small X on top of the cake and insert the chocolate so that they do not show.
6. Cover and microwave again for another 30 seconds until cake fully sets.
7. Place the cake upside down on the plate and allow it to cool before eating.

Plain Biscotti

Nutrition Facts

Plain Biscotti

6 Servings

Amount Per Serving	
Calories	162.6
Total Fat	9.2 g
Saturated Fat	3.7 g
Polyunsaturated Fat	1.1 g
Monounsaturated Fat	2.1 g
Cholesterol	92.5 mg
Sodium	390.0 mg
Potassium	80.8 mg
Total Carbohydrate	12.0 g
Dietary Fiber	2.8 g
Sugars	1.7 g
Protein	11.5 g

These biscotti will fill your requirement for something sweet and sugar-free.

What you need:

½ butter, keep at room temperature
1 tablespoon baking powder
3 cups almond meal
1/4 teaspoon salt
2 eggs
sugar substitute
1 teaspoon vanilla extract
2 teaspoons almond extract

How to prepare:

1. Preheat oven to 350 F. Cover the baking sheet with a parchment paper and grease it will light butter or oil.
2. Mix butter, almond meal, baking powder, salt until they are combined.
3. Add eggs, almond and vanilla extracts, and sugar substitute. Beat all until they are combined.
4. Allow the batter to settle for about 5 minutes to form a dough.
5. Turn the dough to the baking sheet and form it into a rectangle.
6. Bake until you achieve a lightly browned top. This will take about 22-25 minutes. Allow the cookies to cool for 5-10 minutes and cut them into slices measuring 3/4 wide.
7. Place the slices on the sides and place it back in the oven until light brown.
8. Make sure to cool the biscotti completely before storing them.

Brownies

Nutrition Facts

Brownies

12 Servings

Amount Per Serving	
Calories	266.6
Total Fat	21.2 g
Saturated Fat	7.6 g
Polyunsaturated Fat	7.7 g
Monounsaturated Fat	4.9 g
Cholesterol	115.0 mg
Sodium	93.7 mg
Potassium	203.2 mg
Total Carbohydrate	30.7 g
Dietary Fiber	20.9 g
Sugars	6.7 g
Protein	7.4 g

What you need:

1 stick butter

4 eggs

2 cups powdered erythritol

1/2 cup cocoa

1/3 cup cream

2/3 cup water

2 cups flax seed meal

1 tsp. salt

4 oz. melted and unsweetened chocolate

1 tbsp. vanilla

1 tbsp. baking powder

artificial sweetener

optional: 1 cup walnuts

How to prepare:

1. Preheat oven to 350 F and grease a 9 x 13 pan.
2. Cream butter until it becomes fluffy.
3. Mix erythritol and butter until you get a fluffy texture.
4. Add in the vanilla.
5. Add one egg at a time into the mixture and beat well.
6. Add salt and cocoa and beat well.
7. Place the chocolate into the mixture and beat well again.
8. Combine the remaining ingredients.
9. Pour mixture into the pan and bake for 35-40 minutes.
8. Cut into squares.
9. Brownie texture will be different when cooled.

Nutella Fudge

Nutrition Facts

Nutella Fudge

12 Servings

Amount Per Serving

Calories	158.8
Total Fat	4.3 g
Saturated Fat	1.7 g
Polyunsaturated Fat	0.0 g
Monounsaturated Fat	0.1 g
Cholesterol	6.7 mg
Sodium	265.5 mg
Potassium	102.2 mg
Total Carbohydrate	35.5 g
Dietary Fiber	22.7 g
Sugars	9.0 g
Protein	12.6 g

What you need:

4 cups Low Fat Organic Cottage Cheese (880g)
4 tbsp. Psyllium Husk Powder
1½ cups Healthy Homemade Nutella (384g)
1½ tsp. Vanilla-Flavored Stevia Extract
1 cup Powdered Erythritol
1 can Black Beans (15 oz. drained and rinsed)
1/4 cup Cocoa Powder

How to prepare:

1. Blend black beans, Nutella, stevia extract, and powdered erythritol. Blend until completely smooth.
2. Pour the mixture in a large bowl. Sprinkle 1 tablespoon of psyllium husk powder while whisking.
3. Scoop mixture and place in brownie pans. Spread out evenly.
4. Cover with plastic wrap and place in freezer for 3 hours.
5. Remove fudge from brownie pans and slice into pieces.
6. Add cocoa powder and roll the fudge to coat.
7. Place on a serving plate and refrigerate overnight.
*Refrigerating the fudge allows the flavors to meld and improve.

Panna Cotta

Nutrition Facts

Panna Cotta

12 Servings

Amount Per Serving	
Calories	96.6
Total Fat	7.4 g
Saturated Fat	4.6 g
Polyunsaturated Fat	0.3 g
Monounsaturated Fat	2.1 g
Cholesterol	27.3 mg
Sodium	41.3 mg
Potassium	15.4 mg
Total Carbohydrate	7.7 g
Dietary Fiber	0.0 g
Sugars	6.4 g
Protein	1.0 g

What you need:

2 cups of heavy cream

1 envelope of gelatin

1/2 cup of water

1/3 cup of Splenda

How to prepare:

1. Mix ingredients in a small pan.
2. Cook for 10 minutes until mixture thickens.
3. Place cooked mixture in small cups
4. Refrigerate mixture in cups for three hours.
5. Serve cold and enjoy!

Spicy Baked Cauliflower and Sweet Potato

Nutrition Facts

Spicy Baked Cauliflower and Sweet Potato

5 Servings

Amount Per Serving	
Calories	80.7
Total Fat	0.7 g
Saturated Fat	0.1 g
Polyunsaturated Fat	0.3 g
Monounsaturated Fat	0.1 g
Cholesterol	0.0 mg
Sodium	50.2 mg
Potassium	615.7 mg
Total Carbohydrate	17.4 g
Dietary Fiber	5.2 g
Sugars	3.6 g
Protein	3.6 g

This spicy and healthy side dish will add flavor to your meals.

What you need:

4 tbsp. of bacon fat (melted)

2 tbsp. cayenne pepper

1 head of cauliflower (chopped)

1 sweet potato (diced)
1 yellow onion (diced)
1 tbsp. smoked paprika
1 tsp. dried oregano
1 tsp. red pepper flakes
Salt and pepper

How to prepare:

1. Preheat oven to 375°.
2. Add all ingredients in a baking dish. Mix thoroughly.
3. Cook in oven for 35 minutes until sweet potatoes are tender.
4. Serve and enjoy!

Peanut Butter Mousse

Nutrition Facts

Peanut Butter Mousse

12 Servings

Amount Per Serving	
Calories	81.1
Total Fat	7.8 g
Saturated Fat	3.5 g
Polyunsaturated Fat	1.0 g
Monounsaturated Fat	2.6 g
Cholesterol	17.2 mg
Sodium	54.6 mg
Potassium	51.7 mg
Total Carbohydrate	2.8 g
Dietary Fiber	0.3 g
Sugars	0.8 g
Protein	2.1 g

What you need:

4 Ounces of Cream Cheese

1/2 cup of heavy Cream

1 ½ tsp. of Vanilla Pudding Mix

1/4 cup of peanut butter
½ tsp. of Vanilla
1/2 cup of Splenda

How to prepare:

1. Mix heavy cream and vanilla pudding mix into a bowl. Beat the mixture until stiff peaks form.
2. Mix cream cheese and peanut butter in a separate bowl. Microwave it for 20 seconds.
3. Add vanilla and Splenda to the second bowl and whisk until fluffy.
4. Fold whipped cream after
5. Fold the whipped cream in groups until combined.
6. Serve and enjoy!

CHAPTER 5

Quick Snack Ideas and Low Carb Snacks & Beverages

Sometimes, there is a need to eat in-between meals - a bite here and there.

Quick Snack Ideas

If you feel like munching on something but you are too busy to make something else, the list below can be a big help because they do not need any preparation.

1. Hard-boiled eggs
2. Deviled eggs
3. Celery with tuna salad
4. Celery with peanut butter
5. Granola bars
6. Apple with cheese
7. Yogurt
8. Beef or turkey jerky that has low-sugar
9. Nuts
10. Cheese sticks

Beverages

If you feel that you are not much of a water drinker, you can spice up your water and flavor it without worrying about the sugar content. Here are some of the natural ingredients that you can add to your water for a more interesting taste.

1. Lemon or lime
2. Fruit
3. Cucumber
4. Herbal tea bags
5. Any edible flower

Low Carb Snack Recipes

With the recipes below, you do not have to worry about your carbohydrate intake.

The Ultimate LOW CARB Recipes!

Cheese Roll-Ups

Nutrition Facts

Cheese Roll-Ups

5 Servings

Amount Per Serving	
Calories	35.9
Total Fat	2.5 g
Saturated Fat	1.4 g
Polyunsaturated Fat	0.0 g
Monounsaturated Fat	0.0 g
Cholesterol	6.0 mg
Sodium	94.1 mg
Potassium	6.2 mg
Total Carbohydrate	0.6 g
Dietary Fiber	0.3 g
Sugars	0.1 g
Protein	2.9 g

What you need:

2 oz. shredded mozzarella cheese
Garlic powder
Optional: pizza sauce

How to prepare:

1. Heat a 10-inch nonstick pan, place on medium heat and spread the cheese over the entire pan.
2. Sprinkle garlic powder.
3. When the cheese is golden brown, slowly pry it up and roll it.
4. May be dipped in marinara or pizza sauce.

Nachos

Nutrition Facts

Nachos

2 Servings

Amount Per Serving	
Calories	239.5
Total Fat	14.8 g
Saturated Fat	5.5 g
Polyunsaturated Fat	0.3 g
Monounsaturated Fat	0.7 g
Cholesterol	10.0 mg
Sodium	359.7 mg
Potassium	157.5 mg
Total Carbohydrate	24.2 g
Dietary Fiber	3.0 g
Sugars	3.0 g
Protein	5.2 g

What you need:

10 pickled jalapeño slices
1/2 oz. shredded cheddar cheese

How to prepare:

1. Lay the peppers on a single layer on a small plate and top with cheese.
2. Place in the microwave until the cheese melts.

Peanut Butter Protein Balls

Nutrition Facts

Peanut Butter Protein Balls

24 Servings

Amount Per Serving	
Calories	129.2
Total Fat	9.0 g
Saturated Fat	1.7 g
Polyunsaturated Fat	2.2 g
Monounsaturated Fat	4.4 g
Cholesterol	19.2 mg
Sodium	75.0 mg
Potassium	166.1 mg
Total Carbohydrate	4.4 g
Dietary Fiber	1.5 g
Sugars	1.9 g
Protein	9.7 g

What you need:

1 C peanut butter – must be sugar-free
1 1/3 C vanilla or chocolate whey protein powder

1 tsp. vanilla extract

Artificial sweetener

Optional: 1 cup toasted almonds

How to prepare:

1. Mix everything in a mixing bowl.
2. Roll them into balls or on crushed nuts.
3. Place in refrigerator until it becomes firm.

Chocolate Nut Cake

Nutrition Facts

Chocolate Nut Cake

4 Servings

Amount Per Serving

Calories	91.4
Total Fat	6.6 g
Saturated Fat	1.3 g
Polyunsaturated Fat	0.4 g
Monounsaturated Fat	4.6 g
Cholesterol	46.5 mg
Sodium	18.1 mg
Potassium	43.3 mg
Total Carbohydrate	2.8 g
Dietary Fiber	2.1 g
Sugars	0.4 g
Protein	6.4 g

A no-carb dessert if you're craving sweets but want to cut on carbs and sugar.

What you need:

3 tsp. cacao

2 tsp. organic coconut oil

1 whole egg

1 cup Blanched Raw Almond Flour

1/2 tsp. vanilla extract

Organic Stevia

Macadamia nuts

Pinch of salt

Dash of milk

Toppings of your choice

 (Ex. Raspberry &Strawberry)

How to prepare:

1. Mix coconut oil and chocolate powder to create a paste.
2. Add Stevia and a dash of milk. (Depends on how sweet you want it to be)
3. Pour almond flour into chocolate paste. Mix well.
4. Scramble egg and combine in the paste.
5. Bake in oven for 20 minutes.
6. Serve and Enjoy

Shepard's Pie

Nutrition Facts

Shepard's Pie

4 Servings

Amount Per Serving	
Calories	100.8
Total Fat	6.7 g
Saturated Fat	3.6 g
Polyunsaturated Fat	0.2 g
Monounsaturated Fat	1.4 g
Cholesterol	35.0 mg
Sodium	109.7 mg
Potassium	23.8 mg
Total Carbohydrate	1.1 g
Dietary Fiber	0.1 g
Sugars	0.1 g
Protein	9.2 g

What you need:

3 cloves of garlic
1 bay Leaf
1/4 red bell Pepper

Ground turkey
Cheese
Onion Powder
Garlic powder
Onion
Thyme
Salt
Paprika (optional)
Spinach

How to prepare:

1. Cook turkey with the ingredients. Remember to drain of oil when done.
2. Place the turkey at the first layer of a casserole dish. Then add spinach on the second layer. Add cheese on top of spinach.
3. Blend cauliflower and beat until it looks like a mashed potato. Do not add water into the mixture, instead add salt and butter.
4. Spread cauliflower mixture at the next layer.
5. Cover once again in cheese.
6. Bake until the cauliflower and cheese has melted into the pie.
7. Serve and Enjoy!

Black Bean Brownies

Nutrition Facts

Black Bean Brownies

4 Servings

Amount Per Serving	
Calories	89.8
Total Fat	1.2 g
Saturated Fat	0.3 g
Polyunsaturated Fat	0.1 g
Monounsaturated Fat	0.0 g
Cholesterol	0.0 mg
Sodium	23.2 mg
Potassium	159.8 mg
Total Carbohydrate	16.1 g
Dietary Fiber	3.7 g
Sugars	3.7 g
Protein	4.2 g

What you need:

2 tsp. instant coffee or espresso
1 can of black beans
1 box of brownie mix

How to prepare:

1. Rinse the black beans in a colander and return to the washed can.
2. Fill the can with water. Pour in blender until it is smooth.
3. Pour instant coffee, brownie mix, and black bean puree in a large mixing bowl. Mix well.
4. Bake brownies and let cool. Prepare individual servings and enjoy!

Barley-Oat Chocolate Chip Cookies

Nutrition Facts

Barley-Oat Chocolate Chip Cookies

24 Servings

Amount Per Serving	
Calories	82.6
Total Fat	4.2 g
Saturated Fat	0.5 g
Polyunsaturated Fat	2.6 g
Monounsaturated Fat	0.7 g
Cholesterol	22.5 mg
Sodium	12.1 mg
Potassium	58.9 mg
Total Carbohydrate	8.9 g
Dietary Fiber	1.1 g
Sugars	0.7 g
Protein	3.0 g

What you need:

3 tbsp. nonfat dry milk powder

2 eggs

1 cup whole wheat flour

1 cup sugar

1 cup regular rolled oats

1 teaspoon vanilla

1 1/2 teaspoons baking powder

3/4 cup cooking oil

1/2 cup miniature semisweet chocolate pieces

1/2 cup barley flour

1/2 cup chopped walnuts

1/2 cup oat bran

1/4 cup wheat bran

1/4 teaspoon baking soda

1/4 cup unsweetened shredded coconut

How to prepare:

1. Heat oven to about 375 degrees F.
2. Whisk sugar, oil, vanilla and eggs in a medium bowl. Set aside.
3. Combine barley flour, oat bran, whole wheat flour, oats, wheat bran, dry milk powder, baking soda and baking powder in a large bowl.
4. Add the egg mixture to the flour mixture. Stir well until ingredients are combined. Add chocolate pieces, coconuts and walnuts.
5. Place dough into a cookie sheet 2 inches apart. Bake for 10 minutes until all edges are lightly brown.
6. Transfer cookies after baking to a wire rack. Let cool.
7. Serve and Enjoy!

Nutty Carrot Cake Bar

Nutrition Facts

Nutty Carrot Cake

12 Servings

Amount Per Serving	
Calories	114.1
Total Fat	5.1 g
Saturated Fat	0.5 g
Polyunsaturated Fat	3.6 g
Monounsaturated Fat	0.7 g
Cholesterol	0.2 mg
Sodium	7.4 mg
Potassium	71.2 mg
Total Carbohydrate	16.2 g
Dietary Fiber	0.9 g
Sugars	9.2 g
Protein	2.3 g

What you need:

1 1/2 teaspoons pumpkin pie spice
1 cup finely shredded carrot
1 recipe Fluffy Cream Cheese Frosting
1 teaspoon baking powder

3/4 cup all-purpose flour
3/4 cup chopped walnuts or pecans, toasted
1/2 cup sugar
1/3 cup refrigerated or frozen egg product
1/4 cup whole wheat flour
1/4 cup cooking oil
1/4 cup fat-free milk
1/8 teaspoon salt
Nonstick cooking spray

How to prepare:

1. Heat oven to 350 degrees F. Line a foil into a 9x9x2-inch baking pan. Extend the foil over the edges. Coat with nonstick cooking spray. Set aside.
2. Combine wheat flour, sugar, all-purpose flour, pumpkin pie spice, salt and baking powder in a medium bowl. Add carrots, nuts, eggs, milk and oil. Stir well.
3. Pour mixture in the pan. Bake for 20 minutes.
4. Spread top with cream cheese frostings. Sprinkle remaining nuts.
5. Slice, serve and enjoy!

Asparagus Frittata

Nutrition Facts

Asparagus Frittata

6 Servings

Amount Per Serving	
Calories	157.6
Total Fat	11.5 g
Saturated Fat	5.5 g
Polyunsaturated Fat	1.1 g
Monounsaturated Fat	3.9 g
Cholesterol	286.7 mg
Sodium	133.4 mg
Potassium	173.7 mg
Total Carbohydrate	3.1 g
Dietary Fiber	0.5 g
Sugars	0.6 g
Protein	10.9 g

What you need:

6 large eggs
2 tbsp. of butter
1 pound thin spear asparagus (cut diagonally)

1 tbsp. fresh chives (minced)
1 cup Swiss cheese (shredded)
3/4 cup ricotta cheese
1/2 cup sliced shallots
1/2 tsp. of salt
1/4 teaspoon dried tarragon

How to prepare:

1. Heat butter into an oven at medium heat. Cook shallots over until they are soft for about 3 minutes. Add asparagus, stir well.
2. In a bowl whisk ricotta cheese and eggs together. Add chives and tarragon. Pour in the pan with the shallots and asparagus for about 5 minutes.
3. Sprinkle Swiss cheese over eggs and broil until it is brown.
4. Remove pan from oven and serve.

Sports Drink

Nutrition Facts

Sports Drink

1 Serving

Amount Per Serving

Calories	60.0
Total Fat	0.0 g
Saturated Fat	0.0 g
Polyunsaturated Fat	0.0 g
Monounsaturated Fat	0.0 g
Cholesterol	0.0 mg
Sodium	4.7 mg
Potassium	291.5 mg
Total Carbohydrate	23.5 g
Dietary Fiber	1.0 g
Sugars	5.5 g
Protein	1.0 g

Sports drinks have very high sugar content. You can create your own with the following simple mixture:

1 cup water

2 tablespoons lemon juice

a pinch of salt

Flavoring and sweetener to taste

This simple mixture contains the very same amount of potassium found in an 8 oz. sports drink.

To prepare:

Just combine everything in a glass.

Low Carb Iced Coffee

Nutrition Facts

Low-Carb Iced Coffee

1 Serving

Amount Per Serving	
Calories	56.5
Total Fat	5.6 g
Saturated Fat	3.5 g
Polyunsaturated Fat	0.2 g
Monounsaturated Fat	1.6 g
Cholesterol	20.6 mg
Sodium	10.5 mg
Potassium	82.8 mg
Total Carbohydrate	4.2 g
Dietary Fiber	0.0 g
Sugars	0.0 g
Protein	0.5 g

What you need:

1 tablespoon heavy cream
8 oz. cold coffee
1 packet sweetener
a cup of ice cubes

How to prepare:

1. Chill coffee in advance.
2. Combine the chilled coffee, sweetener, and ice cubes.
3. Shake until frothy.

Strawberry Protein Smoothie

Nutrition Facts

Strawberry Protein Smoothie

3 Servings

Amount Per Serving	
Calories	120.0
Total Fat	7.9 g
Saturated Fat	3.8 g
Polyunsaturated Fat	0.5 g
Monounsaturated Fat	2.5 g
Cholesterol	22.3 mg
Sodium	153.0 mg
Potassium	145.7 mg
Total Carbohydrate	12.2 g
Dietary Fiber	2.3 g
Sugars	6.4 g
Protein	2.3 g

What you need:

4 ounces of strawberries
2 ounces cream cheese
2 1/2 cups of cold water
1 tsp. xanthan gum
1 tsp. strawberry extract
2/3 Vanilla flavor powder
1/2 cup sugar free syrup
1/4 cup granular Splenda
Ice cubes

How to prepare:

1. Mix protein powder and xanthan gum in a bowl.
2. Add water, cream cheese, cream, sweetener into a blender.
3. Add the protein powder mixture and again blend briefly.
4. Blend in the highest speed while feeding strawberries through the hole of the blender cover.
5. After adding strawberries, add the ice cubes next. One at a time.
6. Serve and Enjoy!

Iced Frappuccino

Nutrition Facts

Iced Frappuccino

2 Servings

Amount Per Serving

Calories	279.5
Total Fat	29.6 g
Saturated Fat	18.5 g
Polyunsaturated Fat	0.9 g
Monounsaturated Fat	8.7 g
Cholesterol	107.7 mg
Sodium	33.7 mg
Potassium	124.3 mg
Total Carbohydrate	2.6 g
Dietary Fiber	0.0 g
Sugars	0.1 g
Protein	2.0 g

What you need:

4 tbsp. of heavy cream
1 tbsp. of sweetener
1 cup ice
1/2 cup strong brewed coffee
Chocolate syrup
Whipping cream

How to prepare:

Prepare coffee and put in the refrigerator to cool for a couple of hours. Pre-dissolve sugar granules in coffee. Mix cream, coffee, and sweetener in blender. Add ice cubes slowly until the mixture is thick and smooth.
Optional: You can add whipped cream and chocolate syrup as toppings.

CHAPTER 6

Tips in Maintaining a Low Carb Diet

When changing your diet, the most challenging part is to give up the food that you are used to eating regularly. It is not surprising that many people make mistakes when they are first starting with a low carb diet due to the fact that they have been used to eating carbs ever since. Here are helpful tips on what you can do to maintain your diet.

Avoid Going Hungry

Do not deprive yourself of food because the more that you feel hungry, the more that you will want to eat. Do not go hungry. Simply cut down on your calories.

Do Not Eat the Same Food

Eat a variety of foods every day. When you change your diet, it can be very easy to just keep on eating the same food. However, there are a lot of recipes that you can try out to add spice to your diet.

Sleeping Habits

Getting enough sleep is important. Lack of sleep can make your blood sugar level go up.

Follow a Diet that Works for You

Follow your own diet regiment. Do not be bothered about the diet that worked for your neighbor. Each of us has a different body build and nutritional requirements.

Keep Going

Do not give up. There are many ways to low carb dieting. At first, you may encounter some bumps along the way. When everything does not go according to plan, try again.

Stay Away from Junk Food

Low carb snack foods are okay to eat when you are travelling. However, it is a different thing when you make it a part of your daily diet. These low carb bars may have low carbohydrate content but they taste so good that they make you want more.

Get Some Exercise

Exercise is very good for the body. Most people tend to ignore exercise when they are on a low carb diet. One benefit of exercise is that your insulin resistance is lowered. By being consistent with your diet and exercise, you can experience a significant weight loss and keep the weight off.

Would you do me a favor?

I hope this book was able to help you to understand low carb diet more and help you manage your weight in a healthier way.

The next step is to put into application and try out the recipes that are listed in this book.

Finally, if you enjoyed this book, please take the time to share your thoughts and post a positive review on Amazon. It'd be greatly appreciated!

Thank you and good luck!